Nursing & Health Survival Guide

Evidence-based Practice

Judith Davies

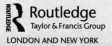

Routledge
Taylor & Francis Group

LONDON AND NEW YORK

First published 2012 by Pearson Education Limited

Published 2014 by Routledge
2 Park Square, Milton Park, Abingdon, Oxon OX14 4RN
711 Third Avenue, New York, NY 10017, USA

Routledge is an imprint of the Taylor & Francis Group, an informa business

Copyright © 2012, Taylor & Francis.

The right of Judith Davies to be identified as author of this work has been asserted
by her in accordance with the Copyright, Designs and Patents Act 1988.

ISBN 13: 978-0-273-74555-6 (hbk)

British Library Cataloguing-in-Publication Data
A catalogue record for this book is available from the British Library

Library of Congress Cataloging-in-Publication Data
A catalog record for this book is available from the Library of Congress

Typeset in 8/9.5pt Helvetica by 35

Printed in the UK by Severn, Gloucester on responsibly sourced paper

MIX
Paper | Supporting
responsible forestry
FSC® C022174

contents

Survival Guide: Evidence-based Practice

Registered nurses must be able to think analytically and use problem-solving approaches and evidence in decision-making (NMC, 2010). Today, regardless of discipline or background, it is accepted that any health care practitioner will function from an evidence-based perspective. The purpose of this text is to provide a guide to utilising an evidence-based framework as a methodology and method for practitioners who seek answers to clinical questions which will ultimately inform and improve practice.

■ EVIDENCE-BASED PRACTICE: WHAT AND WHY?

Definition: 'The conscientious, explicit and judicious use of current best evidence in making decisions about the care of individual patients' (Sackett *et al*., 1997, p. 71).

McKibbon (1998, p. 396) suggests that 'evidence-based practice values, enhances and builds on clinical expertise, knowledge of disease mechanisms and patho-physiology. It involves complex and conscientious decision-making based not only on the available evidence, but also on patient characteristics, situations and preferences'.

Evidence-based practice is about more than the evidence alone. It recognises individual experience, the professional/ client relationship and accepts that clinical decision-making is a complex process which must involve the ethic of caring and doing the right thing by and for the patient.

The terms evidence-based practice and research-based practice are often used interchangeably, but there are fundamental differences. Although both are systematic, they have different purposes. Carnwell (2001) offers a clarification of definitions and purposes in Table 1:

Table 1 Differences between research and evidence-based practice

RESEARCH	EVIDENCE-BASED PRACTICE
Systematic and planned investigation	Systematic search for and appraisal of best evidence
Specification of a problem to be investigated	Use of evidence for making clinical decisions, the evidence often provided by research
Statement of predetermined outcome, e.g. results and recommendations	Account taken of individual needs of the patient, as well as research-based evidence
Contribute to understanding of the world	Bring about changes in practice

The essential difference between research and evidence-based practice appears to be the use of evidence for

ecision-making rather than the creation of evidence through
e research process.

WHAT COUNTS AS EVIDENCE-BASED PRACTICE?

ycroft-Malone *et al.* (2004) stated that evidence is
onsidered to be knowledge derived from a range of sources
at has been broadly differentiated into propositional and
on-propositional or personal knowledge. The formal,
xplicit and generalisable propositional knowledge is derived
om research and scholarship, whereas non-propositional
nowledge is the opposite, being informal, implicit and
erived from and through practice. The tacit knowledge
professionals is otherwise known as professional craft
nowledge (Rycroft-Malone *et al.*, 2004). Knowledge can

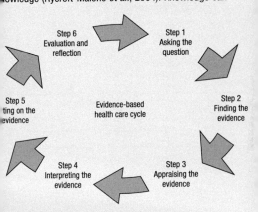

Figure 1 The evidence-based health care cycle

be generated from different types of evidence base for use in clinical practice:

- Research
- Clinical experience
- Patients, clients, carers
- Local context and the environment (Rycroft-Malone *et al.*, 2004).

■ HIERARCHIES OF EVIDENCE

The use of hierarchies of evidence is said to be fundamental in order to distinguish between evidence-based and consensus-based recommendations for practice (Grilli *et al.*, 2000 cited by Spiby and Munro, 2010). A hierarchy simply provides a grading system where the levels of the hierarchy reflect the study design. For example, the National Institute for Health and Clinical Excellence (NICE) offers an authoritative grading system, shown in Table 2:

Table 2 NICE grading system

RECOMMENDATION GRADE	EVIDENCE
A	Directly based on category I evidence
B	Directly based on category II evidence or extrapolated from category I evidence
C	Directly based on category III evidence or extrapolated recommendation from category I or II evidence

able 2 (*continued*)

RECOMMENDATION GRADE	EVIDENCE
)	Directly based on category IV evidence or extrapolated recommendation from category I, II or III evidence
Good practice point	The view of the guideline development group

EVIDENCE CATEGORY	SOURCE
a	Systematic review and meta-analysis or randomised controlled trials (RCTs)
b	At least one RCT
Ia	At least one well-designed controlled study without randomisation
Ib	At least one other type of well-designed quasi-experimental study
II	Well-designed non-experimental descriptive studies, such as comparative studies or case studies
√	Expert committee reports or opinions and/or clinical experience or respected authorities

tional Institute for Health and Clinical Excellence (2003)

The characteristics required by nurses to become evidence-based practitioners are:

- *Observant and sensitive*: look for verbal and non-verbal clues when interacting with patients
- *Empathetic*: develop emotional intelligence, the ethic of caring and recognise patient autonomy
- *Communication*: demonstrate excellence in articulation of knowledge and information-giving to enhance informe patient choice
- *Questioning and challenging practice*: be open to questions in all aspects of practice
- *Reflection in and on practice*: develop critical thinking, new understandings and ultimately clinical decision-making skills
- *Lifelong learning*: keep up to date in ever-changing environments of care and strive continually to improve practice
- *Research knowledge and awareness*: develop a sound understanding of research methodology and critical appraisal of research in order to discriminate between robust or weak evidence (after Cluett and Bluff, 2000).

The six essential steps in the evidence-based practice cycle

STEP 1: ASKING THE QUESTION

The structure is to break down the clinical focus into parts, for example:

	Patient, population or problem
	Intervention
	Comparison
	Outcome

The Centre for Evidence-based Medicine (2006) offers tips for building clinical questions.

Patient/ population/ problem	Starting with the patient, ask how would I describe a group of patients or clients similar to mine? Try and be precise and succinct.
Intervention	Ask which main intervention, prognostic factor or exposure am I thinking of? Be specific.
Comparison	Ask what is the main alternative to compare with the intervention? Be specific.
Outcome	Ask what would I hope to measure or achieve? What can I improve or affect? Be specific.

The benefit of judicious question building is that the search for evidence is easier. Being able to clearly identify and combine the appropriate search terms should make the search for relevant evidence expeditious and simpler. In ord to feel more confident as a practitioner in formulating answerable clinical questions, you will need to practice.

Activity 1

Think of a recent clinical scenario you have encountered.
1. What questions did that scenario give rise to?
2. Try and break down the scenario using the PICO framework
3. Now formulate your patient-focused question

There are alternative frameworks that can be used in trying to build clear and answerable questions. For example:

C	Client group
L	Location
I	Improvement, information or innovation
P	Professionals

E	Expectation
C	Client group
L	Location
I	Impact
P	Professionals
S E	Service

(Wildridge and Bell, 2002)

	Client
	Oriented
	Practical problem
	Evidence
	Search

p://www.evidence.brookscole.com/copes.html

	Setting or context
	Population
	Intervention
	Comparison
	Evaluation

eecroft, Rees and Booth, 2006)

STEP 2: FINDING THE EVIDENCE

nce you have defined your clinical question and broken
down into different elements utilising one of the
ameworks identified, you should be able to identify key
ords which then become your search terms. Hutchfield
010) states there are six elements to a successful
earch strategy:

Selection of the topic
Identification of key words (that best describe the topic)
Focusing the search
Extending or refining the search
Identification of appropriate sources
Keeping an accurate record of the searches

Hart (2001) provides an excellent text on searching for literature. His summary offers a staged approach to a quick search:

Stage 1: familiarise yourself with the library
Stage 2: define your topic
Stage 3: use the quick reference section of the library
Stage 4: search for books in the library
Stage 5: search for articles in journals held by the library
Stage 6: search the Internet (Hart 2001, p. 8)

If you are a novice researcher, you might want to add another stage: enlist the help of a subject librarian. They are knowledgeable about finding sources of information, will guide you through the processes and will probably have tips for locating specific material.

Hart (2001) offers task, tools and outcomes as a useful process in Table 3.

> Remember to keep a log of your searches. The log should provide a transparent account of what you did and you should therefore be able to be replicate it.

■ BOOLEAN OPERATORS

Hart (2001, p. 153) states that in order to search effectively and efficiently online, you will need to employ the use of Boolean logic. This is the logical system of combining words into a statement for searching. For example, using AND, OR, NOT allows you to be more specific and thereby exclude irrelevant literature.

■ REFINING OR KEEPING YOUR SEARCH FOCUSED

You may find that you will have to set inclusion and exclusion criteria when searching for literature. This will ensure an

Table 3 Finding evidence; task, tools and outcomes

TASK	TOOLS	OUTCOMES
Defining the topic	Dictionaries and encyclopaedias	List of key words List of key authors, books and articles
Background knowledge on the topic	Encyclopaedias and textbooks in the library	Initial outline of the topic, key ideas, people and landmarks. Introduction to the vocabulary of the topic
Find sources to consult in order to locate relevant literature	Guides to the literature Subject librarians Internet gateways and directories	List of abstracts, indexes, bibliographies and reference sources
Search for books	Library OPACs* BNB† Publishers' catalogues	List of books with bibliographical details
Search for articles	Indexes and abstracts (electronic and print) Online databases	List of articles with bibliographical details
Search for theses	Dissertation abstracts (electronic and print)	List of dissertations and theses

Table 3 (*continued*)

TASK	TOOLS	OUTCOMES
Search for conference proceedings	Conference proceedings	List of papers in conference proceedings
Search for statistics and official publications	Indexes and abstracts Publishers' catalogues (HMSO)	List of statistical sources and organisations Identification of official publications
Search for grey literature (see p. 15) and research reports	Internet and gateways Research directories	List of items not published List of research reports and organisations
Search for reviews of books and research	Indexes and abstracts Review journals	List of book reviews and evaluations of research
Identify core texts	Citation indexes and bibliographic analysis	Map of the links between publication and highlight landmark studies

*OPAC, Online Public Access Catalogue.
†BNB, *British National Bibliography*.

fective and efficient search strategy in order to maximise
he likelihood of identifying the most relevant literature which
ill ultimately form the core evidence that you seek. Table 4
rovides you with examples of pointers to consider when
ompiling your criteria.

able 4 Example of inclusion and exclusion criteria

INCLUSION	EXCLUSION
• research published within the last 10 years	• research that has been published for more than 10 years
• research published in English	• research not published in the English language
• research published in peer-reviewed journals	• commentaries, editorials or literature that is not based on empirical research
• researchers can be identified	
• researchers are appropriately qualified as experts in their field	• authors of the research cannot be identified
• research discusses ethical considerations and approval processes	• authors of the research appear inappropriately qualified to research the subject
• the title of the research paper reflects its content	• research does not acknowledge ethical considerations
	• the content does not reflect the title of the research

■ SEARCHING FOR EVIDENCE

Hutchfield (2010) usefully identifies key sources of knowledge for evidence-based care, as can be seen in Table 5.

Table 5 Sources of information to support professional practice

SOURCE	EXAMPLE
• Publications from key organisations • Electronic journals • Bibliographic databases • Information gateways • Library catalogues • Professional organisations • News and media • Web 2 technology	• Department of Health • World Health Organization • EBSCO host Electronic Journal Service (EJS) • The Cochrane Library • Pubmed • Cumulative Index to Nursing and Health Literature (CINAHL) • Applied Social Sciences Index and Abstracts (ASSIA) • Intute: www.intute.ac.uk • www.library.nhs.uk • Royal College of Nursing (RCN) • Nursing and Midwifery Council (NMC) • Royal College of Midwives (RCM) • www.bbc.co.uk/health • Blogs, wikis, podcasts (use with caution as the information is not necessarily from reliable sources)

art (2001, p. 94) provides a comprehensive guide on
ow to identify grey literature which is not easily identifiable
r recognised through conventional searching. There are
atabases available which can help you search, for example,
GLE (System for Grey Literature in Europe) and can be
ccessed from some libraries or from SilverPlatter on
D-ROM. Examples of grey literature could include theses,
onference papers, reports, letters, diaries, trade literature
nd fanzines.

Activity 2

Following on from activity one:

1. Plan your search strategy
2. Note your key search terms from your patient-focused/
   research question
3. Carry out your search for evidence
4. Remember to record all of your searches – you might
   want to produce a template or table to record these
   consistently
5. Identify the strengths and limitations of your search
   strategy

NOTE

your search reveals more than 20 or 30 pieces of core
vidence the likelihood is that your research question is too
road. You will need to refine your question so it is more
pecific.

STEP 3: APPRAISING THE EVIDENCE

sing a literature-based study approach, your key or core
vidence becomes akin to the data in primary research.

Before data analysis or synthesis of the findings you must appraise the evidence for its quality, strength, validity and reliability. There are a host of tools available to assist you in this process. First you must immerse yourself in your core evidence. Aveyard (2010) refers to this as 'getting to know your literature'. She suggests there are three assessments you will make during the appraisal process:

1. Is this literature relevant?
2. Have I identified literature at the top of the hierarchy of evidence?
3. Is the literature of sufficient quality to include in my study?

The first step in the appraisal process is to identify what type of evidence you have. At a simple level, identify whether you have qualitative or quantitative evidence, systematic reviews or whether you have information that is not based on research

If you are a novice researcher it is advisable to use a critical appraisal tool, although there has been some debate on the validity of the tools that do exist (Katrak *et al.*, 2004). The aim of the appraisal process is for you to be able to form a judgement about the quality of the evidence you have gathered and to be able to say confidently that it is of good quality and worthy of being included in your study, or that it is of poor quality and should therefore be discarded.

Long (2002) suggests the key criteria for research studies should be:

- Validity – the study was well done and generated good-quality results
- Ethically sound – the study was undertaken according to acceptable and agreed ethical standards and criteria
- Usable – the findings and recommendations are relevant and attainable in clinical practice

Woolliams *et al.* (2009) offer an example of a generic appraisal tool suitable for all types of evidence:

What is being said?

Who is the author?

Why have the authors written this?

How did they carry out their research?

When was it said or written?

Where does the information come from?

Is this evidence relevant to your research topic?

Whilst such a tool may suffice, it possibly lacks sufficient detail to allow an in-depth appraisal. The critiquing tool illustrated in Table 6 is an example of a more detailed approach.

Table 6 Critiquing a research paper

Title
Concise, precise
Authors
Experience, profession
Journal
Accessible, current, peer-reviewed
Abstract
Accurate summary, interesting

QUANTITATIVE	QUALITATIVE
↓	↓

Literature review	
Justification for study	Justification for study
Extensive pre-study	Ongoing
Covers design and tools	

Research topic

Hypothesis/question Dependent and independent variables Extraneous variables	Purpose Aim

↓   ↓

Method

Experimental – surveys Sample size – large Sample selection – probability Inclusion/exclusion criteria Study setting	Grounded theory – phenomenology Sample size – small Sample selection – purposive Describe participants Provide context

Ethical issues

↓

Confidentiality Anonymity Informed consent Access to setting

↓   ↓

Data collection

Duration of study Known tools used Biophysical measurements Structured questionnaires Validity and reliability	Duration of the study Researcher as tool Observation Interviews Trustworthiness

Findings and data analysis

↓	↓
Data collection Raw data in tables and graphs Accurate and matches test Descriptive and inferential statistics Validity and reliability P values, confidence intervals	Transcribing Identification of recurring themes Coding, categorising Descriptive/theory Use of quotes presented with discussion

Discussion

↓	↓
Findings related to literature Research process considered Validity and reliability Limitations identified Generalisability	Literature incorporated Research process reflected on Trustworthiness Limitations Audit trail

Conclusions

↓
Implications for practice Further research

Taken from Cluett and Bluff (2000, p. 194)

There are other resources which have been specifically developed to assist in the appraisal of various levels of evidence. One such resource is that of the Critical Skills Appraisal Programme (CASP) which can be accessed online at http://www.sph.nhs.uk/what-we-do/public-health-workforce/resources/critical-appraisal-skills-programme.

You will find tools for appraisal of systematic reviews, randomised controlled trials, qualitative studies, cohort studies, case-controlled studies, diagnostic test studies and economic evaluation studies. For convenience, these tools have been included in this guide.

Critical Appraisal Skills Programme (CASP) – making sense of evidence

■ TEN QUESTIONS TO HELP YOU MAKE SENSE OF REVIEWS

How to use this appraisal tool

Three broad issues need to be considered when appraising the report of a systematic review:

- Is the study valid?
- What are the results?
- Will the results help locally?

The ten questions are adapted from Oxman AD, Cook DJ, Guyatt GH, Users' guides to the medical literature. VI. How to use an overview. *JAMA* 1994; 272(17), 1367–1371.

SCREENING QUESTIONS	
1. Did the review ask a clearly-focused question? *Consider if the question is 'focused' in terms of:* • The population studied • The intervention given or exposure • The outcomes considered	Yes ☐ Can't tell ☐ No ☐
2. Did the review include the right type of study? *Consider if the included studies:* • Address the review question • Have an appropriate study design	Yes ☐ Can't tell ☐ No ☐

it worth continuing?

DETAILED QUESTIONS	
3. Did the reviewers try to identify all relevant studies? *Consider:* • Which bibliographics databases were used • If there was follow-up from reference lists • If there was personal contact with experts • If the reviewers searched for unpublished studies • If the reviewers searched for non-English-language studies	Yes ☐ Can't tell ☐ No ☐

DETAILED QUESTIONS	
4. Did the reviewers assess the quality of the included studies? *Consider:* • If a clear, predetermined strategy was used to determine which studies were included. Look for: – A scoring system – More than one assessor	Yes ☐ Can't tell ☐ No ☐
5. If the results of the studies have been combined, was it reasonable to do so? *Consider whether:* • The results of each study are clearly displayed • The results were similar from study to study (look for tests of heterogeneity) • The reasons for any variations in results are discussed	Yes ☐ Can't tell ☐ No ☐
6. How are the results presented and what is the main result? *Consider:* • How the results are expressed (e.g. odds ratio, relative risk, etc.) • How large this size of result is and how meaningful it is • How you would sum up the bottom-line result of the review in one sentence	Write comments here . . .

DETAILED QUESTIONS	
7. How precise are these results? *Consider:* • *If a confidence interval were reported, would your decision about whether or not to use this intervention be the same at the upper confidence limit as at the lower confidence limit?* • *If a P value is reported where confidence intervals are unavailable*	Write comments here . . .
8. Can the results be applied to the local population? *Consider whether:* • *The population sample covered by the review could be different from your population in ways that would produce different results* • *Your local setting differs much from that of the review* • *You can provide the same intervention in your setting*	Yes ☐ Can't tell ☐ No ☐
9. Were all important outcomes considered? *Consider outcomes from the point of view of the:* • *Individual* • *Policy-makers and professionals* • *Family/carers* • *Wider community*	Yes ☐ Can't tell ☐ No ☐

DETAILED QUESTIONS	
10. Should policy or practice change as a result of the evidence contained in this review? *Consider:* • *Whether any benefit reported outweighs any harm and/or cost. If this information is not reported can it be filled in from elsewhere?*	Yes ☐ Can't tell ☐ No ☐

■ TEN QUESTIONS TO HELP YOU MAKE SENSE OF RANDOMISED CONTROLLED TRIALS

Three broad issues need to be considered when appraising the report of a randomised controlled trial:

- Is the trial valid?
- What are the results?
- Will the results help locally?

SCREENING QUESTIONS	
1. Did the study ask a clearly-focused question? *Consider if the question is 'focused' in terms of:* • *The population studied* • *The intervention given* • *The outcomes considered*	Yes ☐ Can't tell ☐ No ☐

SCREENING QUESTIONS	
?. Was this a randomised controlled trial (RCT) and was it appropriately so? *Consider:* • *Why this study was carried out as an RCT* • *If this was the right research approach for the question being asked*	Yes ☐ Can't tell ☐ No ☐

it worth continuing?

DETAILED QUESTIONS	
8. Were participants appropriately allocated to intervention and control groups? *Consider:* • *How participants were allocated to intervention and control groups. Was the process truly random?* • *Whether the method of allocation was described Was a method used to balance the randomisation e.g. stratification?* • *How the randomisation schedule was generated and how a participant was allocated to a study group* • *If the groups were well balanced. Are any differences between the groups at entry to trial reported?* • *If there were differences reported that might have explained any outcome(s) (confounding)*	Yes ☐ Can't tell ☐ No ☐

DETAILED QUESTIONS	
4. Were participants, staff and study personnel 'blind' to participants' study group? *Consider:* • *The fact that blinding is not always possible* • *If every effort was made to achieve blinding* • *If you think it matters in this study* • *The fact that we are looking for 'observer bias'*	Yes ☐ Can't tell ☐ No ☐
5. Were all of the participants who entered the trial accounted for at its conclusion? *Consider:* • *If any intervention-group participants got a control-group option or vice versa* • *If all participants were followed up in each study group (was there loss to follow-up?)* • *If all the participants' outcomes were analysed by the groups to which they were originally allocated (intention-to-treat analysis)* • *What additional information would you like to have seen to make you feel better about this?*	Yes ☐ Can't tell ☐ No ☐

DETAILED QUESTIONS	
6. Were the participants in all groups followed up and data collected in the same way? *Consider:* • *If, for example, they were reviewed at the same time intervals and if they received the same amount of attention from researchers and health workers. Any differences may introduce performance bias.*	Yes ☐ Can't tell ☐ No ☐
7. Did the study have enough participants to minimise the play of chance? *Consider:* • *If there is a power calculation. This will estimate how many participants are needed to be reasonably sure of finding something important (if it really exists and for a given level of uncertainty about the final result)*	Yes ☐ Can't tell ☐ No ☐

DETAILED QUESTIONS	
8. How are the results presented and what is the main result? *Consider:* • *If, for example, the results are presented as a proportion of people experiencing outcomes, such as risks, or as a measurement, such as mean or median differences, or as survival curves and hazards* • *How large this size of result is and how meaningful it is* • *How you would sum up the bottom-line result of the trial in one sentence*	Write comments here . . .
9. Were all important outcomes considered? *Consider:* • *If the result is precise enough to make a decision* • *If a confidence interval were reported. Would your decision about whether or not to use this intervention be the same at the upper confidence limit as at the lower confidence limit?* • *If a P value is reported where confidence intervals are unavailable*	Yes ☐ Can't tell ☐ No ☐

DETAILED QUESTIONS	
0. Were all important outcomes considered so the results can be applied? *Consider whether:* • *The people included in the trial could be different from your population in ways that would produce different results* • *Your local setting differs much from that of the trial* • *You can provide the same treatment in your setting* *Consider outcomes from the point of view of the:* • *Individual* • *Policy-maker and professionals* • *Family/carers* • *Wider community* *Consider whether:* • *Any benefit reported outweighs any harm and/or cost. If this information is not reported can it be filled in from elsewhere?* • *Policy or practice should change as a result of the evidence contained in this trial*	Yes ☐ Can't tell ☐ No ☐

■ TEN QUESTIONS TO HELP YOU MAKE SENSE OF ECONOMIC EVALUATIONS

Three broad issues need to be considered when appraising an economic evaluation:

- Is the economic evaluation likely to be usable?
- How were costs and consequences assessed and compared?
- Will the results help in purchasing services for local people?

SCREENING QUESTIONS	
1. Was a well-defined question posed? *HINT: Is it clear what the authors are trying to achieve?*	Yes ☐ Can't tell ☐ No ☐
2. Was a comprehensive description of the competing alternatives given? *HINT: Can you tell who did what to whom, where and how often?*	Yes ☐ Can't tell ☐ No ☐
3. Does the paper provide evidence that the programme would be effective (i.e. would the programme do more harm than good)? *HINT: Consider if an RCT was used; if not, consider how strong the evidence was.*	Yes ☐ Can't tell ☐ No ☐

it worth continuing?

DETAILED QUESTIONS	
. Were all important and relevant resource use and health outcome consequences for each alternative:	Yes ☐ Can't tell ☐ No ☐
a) Identified? HINT: Consider what perspective(s) was/were taken	
) Measured accurately in appropriate units prior to evaluation? HINT: Appropriate units may be hours of nursing time, number of physician visits, years-of-life gained, etc.	Yes ☐ Can't tell ☐ No ☐
c) Valued credibility? HINT: Have opportunity costs been considered?	Yes ☐ Can't tell ☐ No ☐
. Were resource use and health outcomes consequences adjusted for different times at which they occurred (discounting)?	Yes ☐ Can't tell ☐ No ☐
. Was an incremental analysis of the consequences and costs of alternatives performed?	Yes ☐ Can't tell ☐ No ☐

DETAILED QUESTIONS	
7. Was an adequate sensitivity analysis performed? *HINT: Consider if all the main areas of uncertainty were considered*	Yes ☐ Can't tell ☐ No ☐
8. Did the presentation and discussion of the results include enough of the issues that are required to inform a purchasing decision?	Yes ☐ Can't tell ☐ No ☐
9. Were the conclusions of the evaluation justified by the evidence presented?	Yes ☐ Can't tell ☐ No ☐
10. Can the result be applied to the local population? *Consider whether:* • *The patients covered by the review could be sufficiently different to your population to cause concern* • *Your local setting is likely to differ much from that of the review*	Yes ☐ Can't tell ☐ No ☐

TEN QUESTIONS TO HELP YOU MAKE SENSE OF QUALITATIVE RESEARCH

ree broad issues need to be considered when appraising
e report of qualitative research:

Rigour: has a thorough and appropriate approach been
applied to key research methods in the study?

Credibility: are the findings well presented and
meaningful?

Relevance: how useful are the findings to you and your
organisation?

SCREENING QUESTIONS	
. Was there a clear statement of the aims of the research? *Consider:* • *What the goal of the research was* • *Why it is important* • *Its relevance*	Yes ☐ No ☐
. Is a qualitative methodology appropriate? *Consider:* • *If the research seeks to interpret or illuminate the actions and/or subjective experiences of research participants*	Yes ☐ No ☐

Is it worth continuing?

DETAILED QUESTIONS	
Appropriate research design	
3. Was the research design appropriate to address the aims of the research? *Consider:* • *If the researcher has justified the research design (e.g. have they discussed how they decided which methods to use?)*	Write comments here . . .
Sampling	
4. Was the recruitment strategy appropriate to the aims of the research? *Consider:* • *If the researcher has explained how the participants were selected* • *If they explained why the participants they selected were the most appropriate to provide access to the type of knowledge sought by the study* • *If there are any discussions around recruitment (e.g. why some people chose not to take part)*	Write comments here . . .

DETAILED QUESTIONS	
. Were the data collected in a way that addressed the researched issue? *Consider:* • *If the setting for data collection was justified* • *If it is clear how data were collected (e.g. focus group, semi-structured interview etc.)* • *If the researcher has justified the methods chosen* • *If the researcher has made the methods explicit (e.g. for interview method, is there an indication of how interviews were conducted, did they use a topic guide?)* • *If methods were modified during the study. If so, has the researcher explained how and why?* • *If the form of data is clear (e.g. tape recordings, video material, notes etc.)* • *If the researcher has discussed saturation of data*	Write comments here . . .

DETAILED QUESTIONS	
Reflexivity (research partnership relations/recognition of researcher bias)	

6. Has the relationship between researcher and participants been adequately considered?
 Consider whether it is clear:
 • *If the researcher critically examined their own role, potential bias and influence during:*
   – *Formulation of research questions*
   – *Data collection, including sample recruitment and choice of location*
 • *How the researcher responded to events during the study and whether they considered the implications of any changes in the research design*
	Write comments here . . .

DETAILED QUESTIONS	
Ethical issues	
7. Have ethical issues been taken into consideration? *Consider:* • If there are sufficient details of how the research was explained to participants for the reader to assess whether ethical standards were maintained • If the researcher has discussed issues raised by the study (e.g. issues around informed consent or confidentiality or how they have handled the effects of the study on the participants during and after the study) • If approval has been sought from the ethics committee	Write comments here . . .

DETAILED QUESTIONS

Data analysis

| 8. **Was the data analysis sufficiently rigorous?** *Consider:* <ul><li>If there is an in-depth description of the analysis process</li><li>If thematic analysis is used. If so, is it clear how the categories/themes were derived from the data?</li><li>Whether the researcher explains how the data presented were selected from the original sample to demonstrate the analysis process</li><li>If sufficient data are presented to support the findings</li><li>To what extent contradictory data are taken into account</li><li>Whether the researcher critically examined their own role, potential bias and influence during analysis and selection of data for presentation</li></ul> | Write comments here . . . |

DETAILED QUESTIONS	
Findings	
9. Is there a clear statement of findings? *Consider:* • If the findings are explicit • If there is adequate discussion of the evidence both for and against the researcher's arguments • If the researcher has discussed the credibility of their findings (e.g. triangulation, respondent validation, more than one analyst) • If the findings are discussed in relation to the original research questions	Write comments here . . .
10. How valuable is the research? *Consider:* • If the researcher discussed the contribution the study makes to existing knowledge or understanding (e.g. do they consider the findings in relation to current practice or policy, or relevant research-based literature?) • If they identify new areas where research is necessary • If the researchers have discussed whether or how the findings can be transferred to other populations or considered other ways the research may be used	Write comments here . . .

■ TWELVE QUESTIONS TO HELP YOU MAKE SENSE OF A COHORT STUDY

Three broad issues need to be considered when appraising cohort study.

- Are the results of the study valid?
- What are the results?
- Will the results help locally?

The 12 questions on the following pages are designed to help you think about these issues systematically.

SCREENING QUESTIONS	
1. Did the study address a clearly focused issue? HINT: A question can be focused in terms of: • The population studied • The risk factors studied • The outcomes considered • Is it clear whether the study tried to detect a beneficial or harmful effect?	Yes ☐ Can't tell ☐ No ☐
2. Did the authors use appropriate methods to answer their question? HINT: Consider: • Is a cohort study a good way of answering the question under the circumstances? • Did it address the study question?	Yes ☐ Can't tell ☐ No ☐

it worth continuing?

DETAILED QUESTIONS	
3. Was the cohort recruited in an acceptable way? HINT: We are looking for selection bias which might compromise the generalisability of the findings: • Was the cohort representative of a defined population? • Was there something special about the cohort? • Was everybody included who should have been included?	Yes ☐ Can't tell ☐ No ☐
4. Was the exposure accurately measured to minimise bias? HINT: We are looking for measurement or classification bias: • Did they use subjective or objective measurements? • Do the measures truly reflect what you want them to (have they been validated)? • Were all the subjects classified into exposure groups using the same procedure?	Yes ☐ Can't tell ☐ No ☐

DETAILED QUESTIONS	
5. Was the outcome accurately measured to minimise bias? HINT: We are looking for measurement or classification bias: • Did they use subjective or objective measurements? • Do the measures truly reflect what you want them to (have they been validated)? • Has a reliable system been established for detecting all the cases (for measuring disease occurrence)? • Were the measurement methods similar in the different groups? • Were the subjects and/or the outcome assessor blinded to exposure (Does this matter)?	Yes ☐ Can't tell ☐ No ☐
6. (a) Have the authors identified all important confounding factors? List those the authors missed that you think might be important	Yes ☐ Can't tell ☐ No ☐
(b) Have they taken into account the confounding factors in the design and/or analysis HINT: Look for restriction in design and techniques e.g. modelling, stratified, regression, or sensitivity analysis to correct, control or adjust for confounding factors.	Yes ☐ Can't tell ☐ No ☐

DETAILED QUESTIONS	
(a) Was the follow-up of subjects complete enough?	Yes ☐ Can't tell ☐ No ☐
(b) Was the follow-up of subjects long enough? *HINT:* • *The good or bad effects should have had long enough to reveal themselves.* • *The persons that are lost to follow-up may have different outcomes than those available for assessment.* • *In an open or dynamic cohort, was there anything special about the outcome of the people leaving, or the exposure of the people entering the cohort?*	Yes ☐ Can't tell ☐ No ☐
What are the results of this study? *HINT:* • *What are the bottom line results?* • *Have they reported the rate or the proportion between the exposed/unexposed, the ratio/the rate difference?* • *How strong is the association between exposure and outcome (RR)?* • *What is the absolute risk reduction (ARR)?*	Write comments here . . .

DETAILED QUESTIONS	
9. How precise are the results? How precise is the estimate of the risk? *HINT:* • *Size of the confidence intervals*	Write comments here . . .
10. Do you believe the results? *HINT:* • *Big effect is hard to ignore!* • *Can it be due to bias, chance or confounding?* • *Are the design and methods of this study sufficiently flawed to make the results unreliable?* • *Consider Bradford Hills criteria (e.g. time sequence, dose–response gradient, biological plausibility, consistency).*	Yes ☐ Can't tell ☐ No ☐

it worth continuing?

DETAILED QUESTIONS	
1. Can the results be applied to the local population? HINT: Consider whether: • The subjects covered in the study could be sufficiently different from your population to cause concern. • Your local setting is likely to differ much from that of the study • Can you quantify the local benefits and harms?	Yes ☐ Can't tell ☐ No ☐
2. Do the results of this study fit with other available evidence?	Yes ☐ Can't tell ☐ No ☐

One observational study rarely provides sufficiently robust evidence to recommend changes to clinical practice or within health policy decision-making. However, for certain questions observational studies provide the only evidence. Recommendations from observational studies are always stronger when supported by other evidence.

■ TWELVE QUESTIONS TO HELP YOU MAKE SENSE OF A DIAGNOSTIC TEST STUDY

Three broad issues need to be considered when appraising diagnostic test:

- Are the results of the study valid?
- What are the results?
- Will the results help me and my patients/population?

SCREENING QUESTIONS	
1. Was there a clear question for the study to address? *A question should include information about:* • *The population* • *The test* • *The setting* • *The outcomes*	Yes ☐ Can't tell ☐ No ☐
2. Was there a comparison with an appropriate reference standard? *HINT: Is this reference test(s) the best available indicator in the circumstances?*	Yes ☐ Can't tell ☐ No ☐

it worth continuing?

DETAILED QUESTIONS	
. Did all patients get the diagnostic test and the reference standard? *Consider:* • *Were both received regardless of the results of the test of interest?* • *Check the 2 × 2 table (verification bias)*	Yes ☐ Can't tell ☐ No ☐
. Could the results of the test of interest have been influenced by the results of the reference standard? *Consider:* • *Was there blinding?* • *Were the tests performed independently? (review bias)*	Yes ☐ Can't tell ☐ No ☐
. Is the disease status of the tested population clearly described? *Consider:* • *Presenting symptoms* • *Disease stage of severity* • *Co-morbidity* • *Differential diagnoses (spectrum bias)*	Yes ☐ Can't tell ☐ No ☐
. Were the methods for performing the test described in sufficient detail? *HINT: Was a protocol followed?*	Yes ☐ Can't tell ☐ No ☐

Is it worth continuing?

DETAILED QUESTIONS	
7. What are the results? *Consider:* • *Are the sensitivity and specificity and/or likelihood ratios presented?* • *Are the results presented in such a way that we can work them out?*	Write comments here . . .
8. How sure are we about these results? *Consider:* • *Could they have occurred by chance?* • *Are there confidence limits?* • *What are they?*	Write comments here . . .
9. Can the results be applied to your patients/the population of interest? *HINT: Do you think your patients/ population are so different from those in the study that the results cannot be applied? Such as age, sex, ethnicity and spectrum bias.*	Yes ☐ Can't tell ☐ No ☐

DETAILED QUESTIONS	
10. Can the test be applied to your patient or population of interest? Consider: • Think of resources and opportunity costs • Level and availability of expertise required to interpret the tests • Current practice and availability of services	Yes ☐ Can't tell ☐ No ☐
11. Were all outcomes important to the individual or population considered? Consider: • Will the knowledge of the test results improve patient well-being • Will the knowledge of the test results lead to a change in patient management?	Yes ☐ Can't tell ☐ No ☐
12. What would be the impact of using this test on your patients/population?	Write comments here . . .

■ ELEVEN QUESTIONS TO HELP YOU MAKE SENSE OF A CASE-CONTROL STUDY

Three broad issues need to be considered when appraising a case control study:

- Are the results of the study valid?
- What are the results?
- Will the results help locally?

SCREENING QUESTIONS	
1. Did the study address a clearly focused issue? *A question can be focused in terms of:* • *The population studied* • *The risk factors studied* • *Whether the study tried to detect a beneficial or harmful effect*	Yes ☐ Can't tell ☐ No ☐
2. Did the authors use an appropriate method to answer their question? *Consider:* • *Is a case-control study an appropriate way of answering the question under the circumstances? (is the outcome rare or harmful?)* • *Did it address the study question?*	Yes ☐ Can't tell ☐ No ☐

it worth continuing?

DETAILED QUESTIONS	
Were the cases recruited in an acceptable way? *HINT: We are looking for selection bias which might compromise the validity of the findings:* • *Are the cases defined precisely?* • *Were the cases representative of a defined population (geographically and/ or temporally)?* • *Was there an established reliable system for selecting all the cases?* • *Are they incident or prevalent?* • *Is there something special about the cases?* • *Is the time frame of the study relevant to the disease/exposure?* • *Were a sufficient number of cases selected?* • *Was there a power calculation?*	Yes ☐ Can't tell ☐ No ☐

DETAILED QUESTIONS	
4. Were the controls selected in an acceptable way? *HINT: We are looking for selection bias which might compromise the generalisability of the findings:* • *Were the controls representative of a defined population (geographically and/or temporally)?* • *Was there something special about the controls?* • *Was the non-response high? Could non-respondents be different in any way?* • *Were they matched, population-based or randomly selected?* • *Were a sufficient number of controls selected?*	Yes ☐ Can't tell ☐ No ☐

DETAILED QUESTIONS	
. Was the exposure accurately measured to minimise bias? *HINT: We are looking for measurement, recall or classification bias:* • *Was the exposure clearly defined and accurately measured?* • *Did the authors use subjective or objective measurements?* • *Do the measures truly reflect what they are supposed to measure? (Have they been validated?)* • *Were the measurement methods similar in cases and controls?* • *Did the study incorporate blinding where feasible?* • *Is the temporal relation correct? (Does the exposure of interest precede the outcome?)*	Yes ☐ Can't tell ☐ No ☐
. (a) What confounding factors have the authors accounted for? *List others you think might be important, that the authors missed (genetic, environmental and socio-economic)*	Write comments here . . .

DETAILED QUESTIONS	
(b) Have the authors taken account of the potential confounding factors in the design and/or in their analysis? *HINT: Look for restriction in design and techniques e.g. modelling, stratified regression, or sensitivity analysis to correct, control or adjust for confounding factors.*	Yes ☐ Can't tell ☐ No ☐
7. What are the results of this study? *Consider:* <ul><li>*What are the bottom line results?*</li><li>*Is the analysis appropriate to the design?*</li><li>*How strong is the association between exposure and outcome (look at the odds ratio [OR])?*</li><li>*Are the results adjusted for confounding and might confounding still explain the association?*</li><li>*Has adjustment made a big difference to the OR?*</li></ul>	Write comments here . . .

DETAILED QUESTIONS	
. How precise are the results? How precise is the estimate of risk? *Consider:* • *Size of the P value* • *Size of the confidence intervals* • *Have the authors considered all the important variables?* • *How was the effect of subjects refusing to participate evaluated?*	Write comments here . . .
. Do you believe the results? *Consider:* • *Big effect is hard to ignore!* • *Can it be due to chance, bias or confounding?* • *Are the design and methods of this study sufficiently flawed to make the results unreliable?* • *Consider Bradford Hills Criteria (e.g. time sequence, dose–response gradient, strength, biological plausibility)*	Yes ☐ Can't tell ☐ No ☐

Is it worth continuing?

DETAILED QUESTIONS	
10. Can the results be applied to the local population? *Consider whether:* • *The subjects covered in the study could be sufficiently different from your population to cause concern* • *Your local setting is likely to differ much from that of the study* • *Can you estimate the local benefits and harms?*	Yes ☐ Can't tell ☐ No ☐
11. Do the results of this study fit with other available evidence? *HINT: Consider all the available evidence from RCTs, systematic reviews, cohort studies and case-control studies as well for consistency.*	Yes ☐ Can't tell ☐ No ☐

One observational study rarely provides sufficiently robust evidence to recommend changes to clinical practice or within health policy decision-making. However, for certain questions observational studies provide the only evidence. Recommendations from observational studies are always stronger when supported by other evidence.

Activity 3

Utilising an appropriate framework, critically appraise one or more pieces of your core evidence. If you feel you lack confidence in this just keep practising. Critical appraisal is a skill that can be developed.

The critical appraisal process will enable you to make an informed decision about the cumulative quality of your evidence. You will need to summarise your findings and identify collectively what the strengths, weaknesses and limitations of your evidence are.

NOTE

Do not be tempted to 'talk up' the evidence that appears to be of good quality. You need to remain objective and if there appear to be inconsistencies or the evidence lacks consensus, then you must acknowledge this and state this may be difficult to explain.

STEP 4: INTERPRETING THE EVIDENCE

This part of the process is about making sense of the evidence. It concerns the analysis and discussion of key themes that appear to have emerged and been identified from your immersion in the key evidence. Remember that in this methodology, the evidence forms your data.

Analysis is about organising and understanding data (Bluett and Bluff, 2000). In following the evidence-based practice cycle you may find your core (or key) evidence consists of different types of evidence. You could have a systematic review, a randomised controlled trial, a clinical guideline or expert opinion. The art of this part of your study relies on you being able to combine the evidence, and as Aveyard (2010) suggests it is this that makes your literature based study original.

Aveyard (2010) highlights three approaches for summing up the literature.

1. Meta-analysis	• form of research on research • involves statistical analysis of results from a large number of studies • it will only work if combined studies are comparable, i.e. all RCTs • the terms meta-analysis and systematic reviews are used synonymously but classically associated with combining and summarising clinical trials
2. Meta-ethnography	• drawing together a collection of qualitative evidence • involves determining key words, phrases or ideas that occur in some or all of the studies • need to identify connections between studies • identify homogeneity or variance
3. Meta-study	• combining qualitative studies, including underlying theoretical framework, method and data

u might want to think about how you summarise what you
cide will be your key evidence. Producing a template could
 useful. For example, the template in Table 7 is based on
eyard's table.

Assigning codes, developing themes and looking for
atterns is an accepted approach to qualitative data analysis.
is a way of giving meaning to qualitative data (Cluett and
uff, 2000). It is important for you to be able to discuss how
u developed your themes.

Activity 4

ry and develop a cognitive or mind map which illustrates
our themes. You may find that setting out your themes
n diagrammatic format helps you to articulate the links
r relationships between themes. It may also help you
present what appears to be quite complex data in a
impler way.

---

e next step is to determine how closely the codes
d themes relate to your research or clinical question.
 preparation for this, you will probably arrange and
esent your themes in relation to how closely they provide
 answer to your clinical question. Your themes are likely to
 related and therefore should follow sequentially. If some
emes seem incongruent, you must acknowledge this and
ek to explain why this might be.

Table 7 Exemplar: a synopsis of the key evidence

AUTHOR AND DATE	AIM OF THE STUDY	TYPE OF STUDY	THEMES IDENTIFIED	ASSESSMENT OF QUALITY
Peters (2010)	End of life care in the UK	Report of expert committee	Knowledge and skills Training and education Communication and relationships	Methodology robust; large multi-centre sample; good
White (2010)	To explore the lived experience of grief in palliative care nurses	Qualitative	Shared experience Spiritual care and transformation Therapeutic relationships	Inductive; weak
Sinclair (2009)	To evaluate a training programme in advanced communication skills to improve relationships between patients and carers in palliative care settings	RCT	Knowledge and skills Stages of relationships	Large study; sound methodology; good
Black (2007)	To explore nurses' feelings towards breaking bad news to patients	Staff survey	Unpreparedness Grief and loss Therapeutic relationships	Anecdotal evidence; small survey; weak

Each theme should illustrate a different perspective on our argument, thus presenting a holistic and balanced synthesis of information. Hopefully you will have identified an answer to your research question which will be based strong evidence (current best evidence). If your research question has only been partly answered or the evidence is of dubious quality, you must recognise this and will need to make a recommendation for further research studies to be carried out.

In summary, you will now be able to draw together the key issues, highlight the headlines and make some recommendations for future practice.

STEP 5: ACTING ON THE EVIDENCE

Rycroft-Malone and Bucknall (2010), in a series of three texts focusing on the implementation of evidence-based practice, argue that implementing evidence in practice has been overlooked in favour of practitioners developing critical appraisal skills. The significance of implementation is summarised in the next table:

Diffusion	Information is distributed unaided, occurs naturally (passively) through clinicians' adoption of policies, procedures and practices.
Dissemination	Information is communicated (actively) to clinicians to improve their knowledge or skills; a target audience is selected for the dissemination.
Implementation	Actively and systematically integrating information into place; identifying barriers to change, targeting effective communication strategies to address barriers, using administrative and educational techniques to increase effectiveness.
Adoption	Clinicians commit to and actually change their practice.

Source: Adapted from Davis and Taylor-Vaisey (1997). In Rycroft-Malone and Bucknall (2010, p. 6).

A small number of models or theoretical frameworks have been developed to facilitate the implementation of evidence in practice. For example:

OWA model	Titler *et al.* (2001)
ARiHS framework	Kitson *et al.* (1998)
Ottawa model	Graham and Logan (2004)
Stetler model	Stetler (2009) in Rycroft-Malone and Bucknall
Knowledge translation and exchange model (KTE)	Dobbins *et al.* (2005)
Advancing Research and Clinical Practice through Close Collaboration model (ARCC)	Melnyk and Fineout-Overholt (2005)
Joanna Briggs Institute model of evidence-based healthcare (JBI)	Pearson *et al.* (2005)
Knowledge to action framework (KTA)	Graham *et al.* (2006)

Rycroft-Malone and Bucknall (2010, pp. 228–229) suggest that the models and frameworks can be:

Descriptive, in that the model describes the properties, characteristics and qualities of the implementation of evidence into practice

Explanatory, specifying causal relationships and mechanisms of implementing evidence into practice and in relation to other phenomena

Predictive, in that they can predict relationships between the dimensions or characteristics of the implementation of evidence into practice through the hypotheses, for example

	DESCRIPTIVE	EXPLANATORY	PREDICTIVE
Iowa model	✓	✓	
PARiHS framework	✓	✓	✓
Ottawa model	✓	✓	
Stetler model	✓	✓	
KTE model	✓		✓
ARCC model	✓		✓
JBI model	✓		
KTA framework	✓	✓	

Which model will work best for me?

This is difficult to answer because you may choose your model based on what you need it to do unless evidence subsequently emerges that suggests one model is more valid or robust than another. It may be an idea to experiment with different models and not to become a slave to any.

Activity 5

Think about your study themes and how these relate to your clinical question. You should now be able to:
1. Answer your clinical question
2. Draw some conclusions
3. Make some recommendations for clinical practice

Table 8 What will positively influence the implementation of evidence-based practice?

The evidence	For example if it offers benefits to patients or clients, if it is simpler to understand (the more complex the less likely it is to be adopted), if it can be tested out, if clinicians can see others using the evidence, if it can be refined or adapted to suit local need.
Individual clinician	For example, if clinicians can develop critical appraisal skills, can determine validity and reliability of evidence, if they are motivated and open to change.
Health care organisation	For example, the organisation must be receptive to change, willing to take risks or experiment with new evidence. Equally the organisation would be supported by strong leadership, a culture of lifelong learning and a willingness to monitor change, feedback and refine processes.
Communication and facilitation	For example utilising social networks, passionate change champions and use of opinion leaders.
The patient	If patients are enabled to feel included within the decision-making processes, if patient motivation and preferences are respected, their values and beliefs acknowledged.

Adapted from Greenhalgh et al., 2004)

In summary, the following is offered as a framework for this type of study:

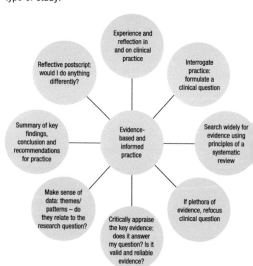

Figure 2 A framework for a literature-based study

■ STEP 6: EVALUATION AND REFLECTION

Your final step in the process of the evidence-based practice cycle utilised in this study guide is an evaluation of whether this step-by-step guide worked for you. The following key questions and final actions should help you to evaluate and complete your study.

Would you use this process or framework again?
Would you modify it in any way? If so, why and how?
What have you learned from this process?
How will you use this learning in your practice?
Freire (1972) suggests that reflection without action is no
ore than wishful thinking. Therefore you must decide how
ur actions will be taken forward.

Activity 6

Formulate an action plan related to the recommendations
that have been highlighted within your study. Consider
publishing your work. Plan to disseminate your findings
within your own organisation or practice environment.

---

o one suggests that this process is easy, but it is essential
at you develop skills and confidence in the process so
u can provide the best possible care for your patients.
e evidence-based health care cycle offers a systematic
pproach for your enquiry. It requires you to be open and
nest about the process followed. Transparency of process
ll strengthen the validity and reliability of the process.
will also say something about you as a researcher or
imary investigator, in that you are cognisant with the
imary ethical principles of respecting autonomy,
neficence and non-maleficence, justice and truth-telling.

   Health care practice will need to be adapted and changed
s new evidence emerges and care environments change. Be
epared, keep informed and when possible work collaboratively
th colleagues from different professional groups. This is
ssential to sustain evidence-based practice, improve health
re and improve outcomes for patients and clients.

References

Aveyard, H. (2010) *Doing a Literature Review in Health and Social Care. A Practical Guide*, 2nd ed. Milton Keynes, Open University Press.

Beecroft, C., Rees, A. and Booth, A. (2006) Finding the evidence. In Gerrish, K. and Lacey, A. (eds) *The Research Process in Nursing*. Oxford, Blackwell, pp. 90–106.

Carnwell, R. (2001) Essential differences between research and evidence-based practice. *Nurse Researcher*, 8 (2), 55–68.

Centre for Evidence-Based Medicine (2006) *Focusing Clinical Questions*. Available from http://www.cebm.net/focus_quest.as

Critical Skills Appraisal Programme (CASP) (2011) *Making Sens of Evidence*. http://www.sph.nhs.uk/what-we-do/public-health workforce/resources/critical-appraisal-skills-programme. Accessed 9 March 2011.

Cluett, E.R. and Bluff, R. (eds) (2000) *Principles and Practice of Research in Midwifery*. London, Bailliére Tindall.

Dobbins, M., Ciliska, D., Estabrooks, C. and Hayward, S. (2005) Changing nursing practice in an organisation. In Dicenso, A., Guyatt, G. and Ciliska, D. (eds) *Evidence-based Nursing: A Gui to Clinical Practice*. St Louis, MO, Elsevier Mosby, pp. 172–20

Evidence-based Practice for the Helping Professions (2011) *Posing a Well-built COPES Question and Classifying it into Or of Five Question Types*. www.evidence.brookscole.com.cope html. Accessed 11 April 2011.

Ellis, P. and Standing, M. (2010) *Evidence-based Practice in Nursing*. Exeter, Learning Matters Ltd.

Freire, P. (1972) *Pedagogy of the Oppressed*. Harmondsworth, Penguin.

Graham, I.D. and Logan, J. (2004) Knowledge transfer and continuity of care research. *Canadian Journal of Nursing Research*, 36 (2), 89–103.

aham I.D., Logan, J., Harrison, M.B., Straus, S., Tetroe, J.M., Caswell, W. *et al.* (2006) Lost in translation: time for a map? *Journal of Continuing Education in Health Professions*, 26 (1), 13–24.

eenhalgh, T., Robert, G., Bate, P., Kyriakidou, O., Macfarlane, F. and Peacock, R. (2004) *How to Spread Good Ideas. A Systematic Review of the Literature on 'Diffussion, Dissemination and Sustainability of Innovations in Health Service Delivery and Organisation'*. London, National Co-ordinating Centre for NHS Delivery and Organisation.

rt, C. (2001) *Doing a Literature Search*. London, Sage.

tchfield, K. (2010) Sources of knowledge for evidence-based care. In Ellis, P. and Standing, M. *Evidence-based Practice in Nursing*. Exeter, Learning Matters Ltd, pp. 21–35.

trak, P., Bialocerkowski, A.E., Massey-Westropp, N., Kumar, S. and Grimmer, K.A. (2004) A systematic review of the content of critical appraisal tools. *BMC Medical Research Methodology*, 4 (22), 22–33.

tson, A.L., Harvey, G. and McCormack, B. (1998) Enabling the implementation of evidence-based practice: a conceptual framework. *Quality in Health Care*, 7 (3), 149–158.

ng, A.F. (2002) Critically appraising research studies. In McSherry, R., Simmons, M. and Abbott, P. (eds) *Evidence-Informed Nursing. A Guide for Clinical Nurses*. London, Routledge, pp. 41–64.

cKibbon, K.A. (1998) Evidence-based practice. *Bulletin of Medical Library Association*, 86 (3).

elnyk, B.M. and Fineout-Overholt, E. (2005) *Evidence-based Practice in Nursing and Healthcare. A Guide to Best Practice*. Philadelphia, PA, Lippincott, Williams and Wilkins.

National Collaborating Centre for Women's and Children's Health (2008) *Antenatal Care: Routine Care for the Healthy Pregnant Woman*. London, RCOG Press. Available from www.nice.org.uk/CG062fullguideline.

NMC (Nursing and Midwifery Council) (2010) *Standards for Pre-registration Nursing Education*. London, Nursing and Midwifery Council.

Pearson, A., Wiechula, R., Court, A. and Lockwood, C. (2005) The JBI model of evidence-based healthcare. *International Journal of Evidence-based Healthcare*, 3 (8), 207–215.

Rycroft-Malone, J. and Bucknall, T. (eds) (2010) *Models and Frameworks for Implementing Evidence-Based Practice*. Chichester, Wiley-Blackwell/Sigma Theta Tau International.

Rycroft-Malone, J., Seers, K., Titchen, A., Harvey, G., Kitson, A. and McCormack, B. (2004) What counts as evidence in evidence-based practice? *Journal of Advanced Nursing*, 47 (1), 81–90.

Sackett, D.I., Richardson, W.S., Rosenberg, W. and Haynes, R.B. (1997) *Evidence-based Medicine. How to Practice and Teach EBM*. Edinburgh, Churchill Livingstone.

Spiby, H. and Munro, J. (eds) (2010) *Evidence-based Midwifery. Applications in Context*. Chichester, Wiley-Blackwell.

Titler, M.G., Kleiber, C., Steelman, V.J., Rakel, B.A., Budreau, G. Buckwalter, K.C. *et al.* (2001) The Iowa Model of evidence-based practice to promote quality care. *Critical Care Nursing Clinics of North America*, 13 (4), 497–509.

Wildridge, V. and Bell, L. (2002) How CLIP became ECLIPSE: a mnemonic to assist in searching for health policy/management information. *Health Information and Libraries Journal*, 19 (2), 113–115.

Woolliams, M., Williams, K., Butcher, D. and Pye, J. (2009) *Be More Critical. A Practical Guide for Health and Social Care Students*. Oxford, Oxford Brookes University.